YOUR KNOWLEDGE HAS VALUE

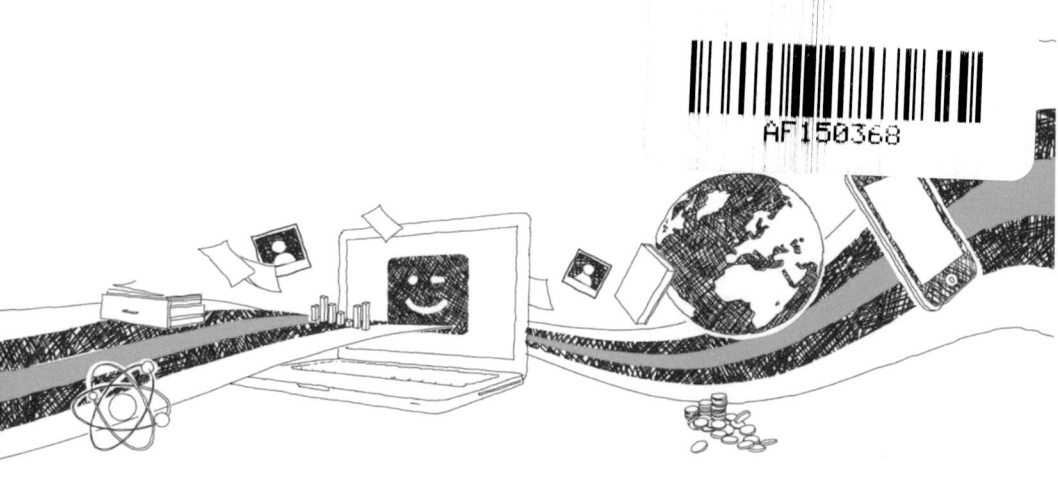

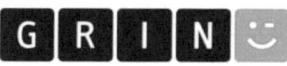

Muhammad Kamran Taj, Taj Muhammad Hassani, Imran Taj, Rehan Jamil, Irfan Jamil, Ashfaq Ahmed, Wei Yunlin

Research Report on Community Livestock Workers in Balochistan

GRIN Publishing

Bibliographic information published by the German National Library:

The German National Library lists this publication in the National Bibliography; detailed bibliographic data are available on the Internet at http://dnb.dnb.de .

Imprint:

Copyright © 2014 GRIN Verlag GmbH
Print and binding: Books on Demand GmbH, Norderstedt Germany
ISBN: 978-3-656-62377-9

This book at GRIN:

http://www.grin.com/en/e-book/270758/research-report-on-community-livestock-workers-in-balochistan

GRIN - Your knowledge has value

Since its foundation in 1998, GRIN has specialized in publishing academic texts by students, college teachers and other academics as e-book and printed book. The website www.grin.com is an ideal platform for presenting term papers, final papers, scientific essays, dissertations and specialist books.

Visit us on the internet:

http://www.grin.com/

http://www.facebook.com/grincom

http://www.twitter.com/grin_com

Research Report on Community Livestock Workers in Balochistan

Muhammad Kamran Taj[1], Taj Muhammad Hassani[2], Imran Taj[3], Rehan Jamil[4], Irfan Jamil[5], Ashfaq Ahmed[6] and Wei Yunlin[7]

[1,6,7]Kunming University of Science and Technology, Yunnan, China
[2]Food and Agriculture Organization, Balochistan, Pakistan
[3]Centre for Advanced Studies in Vaccinology and Biotechnology, UoB Balochistan, Pakistan
[4]School of Energy & Environmental Science, Yunnan Normal University, Kunming, China
[5]College of Energy & Electrical Engineering, Hohai University, Nanjing, China

INTRODUCTION:

Existing government line department services are mainly focused upon providing veterinary service to hardly 11 to 14% livestock of the province. In order to narrow the existing gape in the provision of animal health care services and to cater farmer's need for improved livestock production technologies there is need to develop community based extension services. Good results with such approach were achieved by Mercy Crop International in Afghanistan and by European Economic Commission (EEC) & Asian Development Bank (ADB) assisted Balochistan livestock department projects in some parts of the province.

Since past decade there has been gradual shift in provision of animal health services towards community manage extension services because of UN agencies and other international donors started involving communities in this task. This concept eventually leads to evolution of professionally trained sustainable service providers.

With the liberalization of animal health services in Balochistan, community livestock extension workers (CLEWS) have become an important alternative animal health delivery channel in the Balochistan's marginal areas.

Lack of empathy between the extension staff , particularly the urban based veterinary officers and ordinary rural people and a poor understanding by the technically trained extension workers about the real life situation in the rural areas.

Center for Advanced Studies in Vaccinology and Biotechnology (CASVAB) University of Balochistan developed a comprehensive training module and gave training to CLEWS of Balochistan Rural Support Program and IUCN. 40% of trained CLEWS have begun earning their livelihood. On average Rs. 2500 to 3000 per month is being earned by each CLEW working in his village.

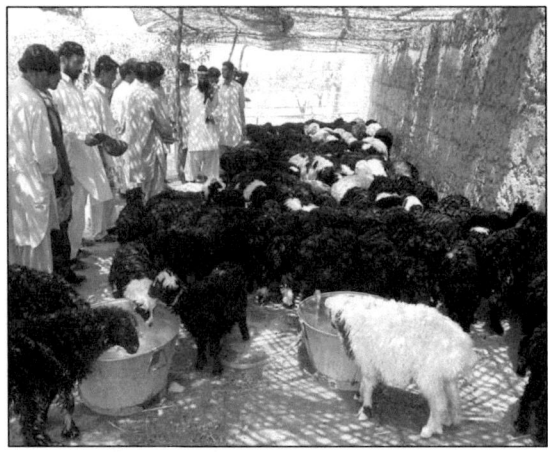

This initiative involves training farmers and community representatives in basic animal health and production techniques. They are taught about deferent small livestock businesses such as home poultry, dairy farming, animal nutrition, basic surgery, milk production management.

Multilinguecy and socio-cultural differences after every 50 to 80 miles, limits the free approach, particularly of urban based supervisors to most rural parts of the province. Therefore it is of paramount importance to select people for extension services with a farming background, from rural areas having real empathy with their fellow farmers

SELECTION OF CLEWS:

The procedures and criteria for selection trainees are crucial to their success and sustainability.

CLEWS are selected by community .The degree of democracy in the process varies according to the cultural and social content .Local socio-political division exist in many rural communities and village hierarchies and are not easily by passed, thus creating problem in fare selection.

Personal characteristic of candidates are the hardest to define and measure but are critical, towards sustained support and respect within a community.

Among other criteria literacy is seen as a prerequisite for learning and drug handling activities, but there are many evidences, however that illiterate trainees can be trained equally effectively.

Gender remains a sensitive issue, since it is apparent that communities tend to have a male bias in the selection of trainees. There is little discussion of why this should be, although many programmes actively discuss the important role of women in raising livestock and their potential as CLEWS candidates.

MONTORING AND EVALUATION OF CLEWS:

The importance of monitoring and evaluation of impact on the results of CLEWS programmes are essential for the sustainability of approach. Monitoring covers the use of programme resources, the numbers and content of training programme and subsequently recording of the basic CLEWS activities and clientele.

TRAINING STRUCTURE AND DURATION:

Training structure and its contents are vital factors in clews programme. The technical content and scheduling of training course should be planned in the context of local farming system. Theoretical and practical training of 4 to 6 weeks is usually sufficient to professionally harness the CLEWS.

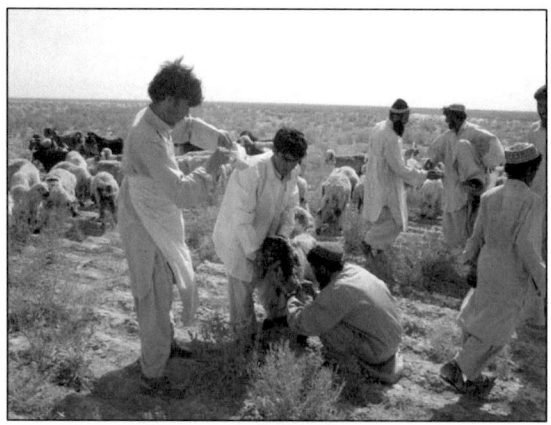

The CLEWS training package should include identification, diagnosis and treatment of all common livestock diseases, the handling and use of veterinary medicine and vaccines, production techniques, extension skills, food hygiene, produce marketing and business with sound management skills.

ACKNOWLEDGEMENTS:

I am very thankful to CASVAB UoB, for providing financial support for this study. I would also like to express my very great appreciation to Professor Shakeel Babar and Ferhat Abbass, for their valuable and constructive suggestions during the planning and development of this work.

picture-© by the authors